You Were Healed

I Peter 2:24

by Eric Holzapfel

PushButtonPress.com, Inc. U.S.A.

<u>**You Were Healed**</u>
By Eric Holzapfel

Except for brief quotations, written permission is required to reproduce any portion of this book.

Publisher's Note Regarding Responsibility of the Material in this Book:

"Congress shall make no law respecting an establishment of religion, or prohibiting the free exercise thereof; or abridging the freedom of speech, or of the press; or the right of the people peaceably to assemble, and to petition the government for the redress of grievances."

- First Amendment to the Constitution of the United States of America.

"But these are written, that ye might believe that Jesus is the Christ, the Son of God; and that believing ye might have life through his name."

-John 20:31 (KJV) -

"How beautiful upon the mountains are the feet of him that bringeth good tidings, that publisheth peace; that bringeth good tidings of good, that publisheth salvation; that saith unto Zion, 'Thy God reigneth!'"

Isaiah 52:7 (KJV) -

As the publisher, I have published good news on this page to bring God's blessings. The author is responsible for the contents of the rest of this book. As a lover of freedom, I encourage the author's right to say their peace. As the reader, you are responsible for the wise application to your life of anything in this book.

Sincerely,

Donald Kubelka
Publisher
PushButtonPress.com, Inc.

"If I do not the works of my Father

believe me not.

But if I do,

though ye believe not me

believe the works..."

- John 10:37-38 -

Dedication

This book is dedicated to all those who desire to know more fully the Lord Jesus Christ.

Many thanks to Donald Kubelka, Timothy Fraher, Dan Kubelka, Edward Zahigian, and many others who have helped me to put this book together.

May the Lord Jesus be glorified throughout this work!

"Who his own self bare our sins

in his own body on the tree,

that we,

being dead to sins,

might live unto righteousness,

by whose stripes you were healed."

- 1 Peter 2:24 -

Contents

*"And these signs shall follow them
that believe.*

*in my name they will cast out
devils;*

they shall speak with new tongues;

they shall take up serpents;

*and if they drink any deadly thing,
it shall not hurt them;*

*they shall lay hands on the sick
and they will recover."*

- Mark 16:17 -

Introduction

"Whether it is easier, to say, Thy sins be forgiven thee; or to Say, rise up and walk?"

~Luke 5:23 -

Have you ever wondered why many people don't get healed, even after they have received prayer?

And many Christians have fallen sick and died.

Why is this?

Why do we fear sickness?

Do you happen to know someone who is suffering with it?

What is God's will concerning the sickness?

Can we really trust the Bible as the Word of God?

These questions, and more, I will endeavor to answer as you continue reading this book.

The following is an account of my own experience as regards to the ministry of the Holy Spirit and God's healing virtue:

It began in the summer of 1984, when our church in Dusseldorf, Germany, was visited by two evangelists from the United States.

This dear elderly couple came to us with the good news of the baptism of the Holy Spirit.

Their message had had a marvelous effect in every church that they had visited.

It was not unusual for us to have special speakers because our pastor was always very eager for those under his care to receive the very best teaching. As a result, the church has for years remained a meeting place for people from all Christian denominations.

On the very first day of their visit, I personally believed on the Lord Jesus for the reality of the Holy Spirit baptism. Consequently, I began to speak with tongues in the same manner as is reported in the early church of the book of Acts.

At that very same moment I experienced, through this personal encounter with my Heavenly Father, a filling of power. **It was a power that literally felt like it was running through my veins.**

I wept for a good five minutes, and remembered the scriptures in the Bible that talked about the peace that passed all understanding. That was certainly it!

Afterwards, I felt even more strongly that my Heavenly Father loved me with great compassion, grace, and love.

During that same period of time, I had been suffering from severe migraine headaches; sometimes twice a week.

To my relief, the Father sent another man of God who, at that time, shared with me the *healing power of Jesus*. He took my hand and thanked the Father for sending Jesus to heal me.

From then on, I experienced no further attacks!

I even tested it by eating everything that would normally activate the migraines, and yet had no ill effects.

On that same day, I asked the minister a question. "Could I pray for the sick?"

His reply was simply that I should ask the Father.

So I did, and from that moment on, I had an unusual thirst for reading and meditating on every scripture that concerned healing.

A month later, I asked God to use me for healing the sick.

Strangely enough, shortly after that prayer I and some others were invited to pray for a six month old child. The baby was the granddaughter of an Anglican pastor, and she had a malignant cancerous tumor behind her right eye.

The pastor instructed those who were present to lay hands on the child according to the scriptures and we asked God to heal and remove the tumor.

After the laying on of hands, the child was checked by a physician, but the tumor was still visible and dangerous.

Some time later, specialists were flown in and said that the child's eye would have to be removed to even get at the tumor.

However, several days after the laying on of hands, I was asking the Father why our prayers didn't work right away.

I had been healed immediately, and the Bible says that we "were" healed, (past tense).

As I was praying, I heard an answer that surprised me. **"I know you Eric, and I know full-well that if you really believed that the child was healed, you would be the first to tell everyone. But, you have kept silent... in fear, just in case. This is not faith, but hope."**

I happened to be driving to work while I was having this conversation with God and asked that inner voice, which I know to be the Holy Spirit, "what must I now do if I did believe?"

The reply was to phone the mother of the child as soon as I arrived at my business, and tell her what I believed and why I believed it.

I trembled at the thought of what could go wrong if what I was hearing was only my imagination.

The child was the granddaughter of a pastor who visited us regularly! His wife was even a good friend of my wife, Angelika, and there seemed to be so much to lose.

However, I weighed it in comparison with the child's life. I finally surmised that relationships come and go, and can always be repaired, but the child herself had only one life to live.

When I arrived at my business I called the mother of the child and told her **that her baby was healed**, and that I was speaking in the name of the Lord Jesus Christ.

She received my message and answered that she would love to believe what I told her, but...

That was when I told her that it was, **"written in the Holy Scriptures, and that she only had to trust God."**

I also asked her if the physicians gave her any guarantee of success...

That was on a Friday, and by the following Monday the operation was to take place.

Monday came and my wife accompanied the mother and child to the hospital where the specialist told them that they could not guarantee anything, and that they might have to take out the second eye as well.

At the bitter news, the child's mother refused the operation and **decided to trust in the Bible.**

If I may, I'd like to affirm here that the Word of God is still as powerful today as it was nearly two thousand years ago when the disciples were experiencing miracles and healing on a daily basis.

The wonderful words: ***"By His Stripes*** (wounds on Jesus' body) ***you were healed,"*** (1 Peter 2:24) and ***"He took our pains and carried our sicknesses,"*** (Matthew 8:17), still remain powerful for those who decide to trust in them with their whole heart, soul, mind, and strength.

When we trust and rely upon His words, we are trusting in Him and in His power to perform them.

"Only believe", Jesus said to His followers and that is exactly what that little child's mother decided to do!

The child was healed and her beautiful blue eyes remained untouched.

Praise God!

The physicians had no explanation for the healing.

Jesus had not changed, for He was, and is, still the Lord who heals us!

I have shared this true story with you to help you realize that first and foremost, God's Word is the truth.

Secondly, I would like you to know that God still uses believers young and old for His glory. **They just need to know His will, which is in the Word of God, and then act upon it.**

As we continue together, we will learn to do just that. One simple step of faith at a time. So join me as we journey into the wonderful world of God's miraculous healing power where...

You were healed!

"Behold,

now is the accepted time;

behold,

now is the day of salvation."

- 2 Corinthians 6:2 -

<u>*Chapter One*</u>

Becoming a Child of God

"Did I not say to you that if you would believe you would see the glory of God?"

- John 11:40 -

The Bible tells us in Romans 10:9 that, *"if you confess with your mouth the Lord Jesus and believe with your heart that God raised Him from the dead, you will be saved."* With these words and others, we trust God for the salvation of our souls and are born of God.

The Apostle John tells us in his letter to the believers: *"Whoever believes that Jesus is the Christ, (the Anointed One), is born of God."* (1 John 5:1).

The Apostle Peter said, *"having been born again (we who believe are made) not of corruptible seed, but incorruptible through the word of God, which lives and abides forever."* (1 Peter 1:23).

Therefore, **you are no longer limited to natural resources.** In Jesus' name you can walk in heavenly places and share in the power of God.

You are accepted and loved by the Creator of the Universe. He calls you His sons and daughters and forgets all your failures, and He gives you the power to be like Him... to even rule with Him!

It's what we call, "The good news... the gospel."

Before you read any further, I would like you to ask yourself if you truly believe that the Holy Bible is the perfect Word of God.

If you are doubtful, just ask God in Jesus' name to reveal the truth to you. He will answer.

In fact, with a sincere and simple prayer, the Holy Spirit Himself will reveal what God means in His eternal Word.

The following prayer is based on Romans 10:9 and Acts 1:8. It will lead you to be born into the Kingdom of God and become his son or daughter.

So, if you are ready, pray like this:

"Heavenly Father, I believe that Jesus is Lord, and that He died for my sins and rose from the dead on the third day as it is written in your Word.
Holy Spirit, please empower me to be a good witness, and help me to receive all of your precious promises.

Thank you Jesus for saving and healing me.

I renounce the devil... Satan, I bind you in the name of Jesus, now! Get out of my life!

In the name of Jesus Christ I am set free. Amen"

Now that you have prayed the prayer of faith, go and tell someone of your decision to follow Christ.

With this, we can go on for the glory of Jesus.

You have the Holy Spirit in you, the Word of God (Jesus), and the love of the Father. We are the temple (His body), and He dwells in us so that He might rule and reign here on earth. (John 14:23).

Your decision has opened a door for you. A door that no one can shut.

You can now enter the wonderful Kingdom of Heaven and experience the love of your Heavenly Father. (Col. 1:13)

Jesus said, *"I am the way, the truth, and the life and no one comes to the Father except through me."* (John 14:6). And again He says that, *"I am the door."* (John 10:9)

Follow Him, listen to Him, and live by Him.

There are so many beautiful things happening in the Kingdom of God and I welcome you to God's wonderful Kingdom where miracles are an everyday affair.

To further encourage you, I would like to share an incident that I was involved in.

Some time ago, an antique dealer walked into a business that I was managing. She had "just popped in" to look around.

While I was talking to her, I received a <u>word of knowledge</u> concerning her health. The word was **that she was dying**.

(Thank God that I had shared what God had told me then. Had I waited, the results could have been disastrous.)

I let her know that the Jesus who was in me loves her, and **wanted to heal her right then and there.**

After some sharing, the lady asked for prayer because of the pain she was experiencing.

I told her that the scriptures assure us that, *"we who believe,"* will lay hands upon the sick, and they shall recover.

Then I asked her if she would allow me to do this.

She did.

After the laying on of hands and a prayer of faith, I asked her if the pain had left.

She confirmed that it did, and even added that she felt power coming from my hands and a warmth that permeated the area that pained her!

Praise God!

She was a Jewish lady and did not yet declare Jesus as her Lord, but she knew that something wonderful had just happened.

The death that I saw in her eyes was no longer there.

I assured her that whatever she suffered from was gone.

Some days later she confirmed the word that I got from God and told me that she was diagnosed with cancer of the lungs and the doctors had given up on her.
However, tests showed the cancer in remission.

She then wanted to know more about my faith and what I based it on.

Therefore, I led her to the Bible and within a month that Jewish art dealer believed in Jesus Christ as her Messiah and Lord.

What a great God we love and serve for He is still the "living God." The God of Abraham, Isaac, and Jacob!

Chapter Two

God's Word is God's Will

"For the Word of God is quick, and powerful, and sharper than any two-edged sword... "

- Hebrews 4:12 -

How am I so confident that you can receive the healing of Jesus right now?

It is by the Word of God, the Holy Bible, and through personal experience.

It is also through the testimonies of others.

You see, once we have dedicated our lives to Jesus for the salvation of our souls, everyone of us can trust upon His Word and have the confidence that He is also able to perform healing.

So, what am I stating when I proclaim that God's Word is God's will?

Well, in short, the Bible is made up of the Old and New Testaments...

Just as in our everyday lives, we clearly understand that when a relative leaves us something in their will, we will most certainly receive it.

It is the will that speaks for the deceased person even after their death. Their will and testament states their desire to bless the other family members.

Therefore, the New Testament, which supersedes the Old, is the will and testament of God to bless His sons and daughters, His heirs. That is, you and I, who believe and trust in Jesus Christ as our Lord and Savior.

Hebrews, chapter eight explains that God designed, *"a better covenant with better promises,"* and that, *"the new covenant"* (New Testament) **has made the first obsolete.**

The term "Old Testament" refers to the will, or covenant between God and the Jewish people.

This will continued until Jesus sealed the new covenant with the shedding of His blood and consequential death on the cross.

The New Testament, from Matthew to the Revelation, is therefore a written will from God to us through Jesus Christ.

Thus, God's Word is God's will.

The Word of God is our inheritance!

If we are left a will or testament by our parents, do we not read every word of the document to make sure that we get everything that is coming to us?

I remember that long ago I was included in a family will. Upon receiving a copy of the document, at the death of a relative, **I read it again and again and again until I had almost every word memorized.**

I was determined to know what was coming to me. I made sure that on the day of payment, I received everything that was rightfully mine.

However, **I only believed it after reading it over and over.**

(By the way, I was still thinking in a very worldly manner at the time.)

Likewise, you and I must read the testament that our Father **left to us through Jesus. We should read it again and again.**

If we are ignorant to what is promised to us, we will most likely be cheated out of our inheritance by the devil. He is the one that will try to deceive us and keep us from our inheritance **because he knows that we have been given the authority and power to rule and reign here on earth as sons and daughters of God.**

A lot of what we have inherited has been taken by Satan.

The Bible tells us that the devil is like a roaring lion, roaming around seeking whom he may devour.

All of us must be diligent when it comes to the Word of God and **take back what he stole from us and our forefathers.**

The discipline of reading the Bible daily is probably the best way to remain free and clean from all evil schemes set up to bind us and render us powerless.

The devil uses false doctrines to confuse us so that fear can enter our minds. Satan knows that the power of fear can keep us immobile long enough for him to cause his evil desires to materialize.

Reading the Bible defeats the false doctrines that have been implanted into our minds, and thus, sets our minds free from fear and doubt.

Remember, ***"the word is living and powerful,*** *and sharper than any two-edged sword piercing even to the division of soul and spirit, and of joints and marrow, and is a discerner of the thoughts and intents of the heart."* (Hebrews 4:12).

Don't forget, the Word of God is still as powerful today as it was nearly two thousand years ago, when the first disciples of Jesus were experiencing daily miracles and healing.

Let's read together some of this precious document that is sealed by the blood of Jesus and the power of the Holy Spirit.

The gospel of John begins with these words: *"In the beginning was the Word, and the Word was with God and **the Word was God... And the Word became flesh** and dwelt among us..."* John 1: 1,2,14).

Yes, the Word of God became flesh and walked among us and we know Him as Jesus Christ the son of God.

If you and I believe that this passage is the Word of God, then we can also be sure that God's Word, (His son) sustains us, and without this Word we would not even exist.

Some people have a rebellious and unbelieving heart and discard the Bible, discrediting it by calling it mere literature.

But I say to them in Jesus' name, "Everything that contradicts the scriptures and the healing power of the Bible is from the devil."

Those who choose to believe and trust the Bible must accept all of God's Word as divinely inspired. (2 Timothy 3:16).

Why do all the cults and philosophies of men always try to discredit the Bible?

Because, if they can cause their fellow man to doubt the Bible, then no one will be able to claim their inheritance and the devil will take it by default.

However, through faith we can defeat those plans and receive all that God has prepared for us, **but if we doubt we should expect nothing.** (James 1:6,7)

We can truly trust in the Bible to be God's will for us.

That is, **we who believe in Jesus Christ.**

Thank God that we have a strong foundation in this world of trouble.

I encourage you to receive the Bible as a love letter from God. Along with this love letter, He has enclosed His will and testament. Read it and in the name of Jesus, live every word to its fullest.

I also want to encourage you to read the Bible on a daily basis.

Get to know Jesus, the Father, and the Holy Spirit, for you will surely experience the heavenly kingdom here on earth.

Instead of being motivated by fear, you will rise up in faith and conquer all of your fears.

You will also learn how to trust and love your Creator and do wonderful feats in His name. Embrace these truths and embrace the great destiny that is stored up for you in the kingdom of our God and Father.

Embrace them in the name of Jesus!

"For God hath not given us

the spirit of fear;

but of power,

and of love,

and of a sound mind."

- 2 Timothy 1:7 -

<u>*Chapter Three*</u>

Knowledge Over Fear

"There is no fear in love; but perfect love casts out fear, because fear involves torment. But he who fears has not been made perfect in love."

- 1 John 4:18 -

Lack of knowledge is a sorry thing.

Through ignorance we suffer pain, illnesses, and separation from God... and then many times, we blame God for them all.

What a terrible situation.

The saying that comes immediately to mind is: *"My people are destroyed for lack of knowledge."* (Hosea 4:6)

But... we don't have to stay in that condition!

We are told to read God's Word, and to meditate on the scriptures daily.

Proverbs 4:22 states that the Word of God is life and health to the flesh of those who find it.

It is the ignorance that separates us from the promises of God.

However, we are also told that it is by grace, through faith, that we are saved. (Ephesians 2:8).

How can we be saved if no one tells us the way of salvation?...

Easy, knowledge!

The book of Romans reminds us that we were all given a conscience to know good and evil, and that even creation itself portrays the wonders of God.

But, we have all fallen from grace and no longer have the power to return to God without the blood of Jesus.

Jesus is the only way back to fellowship with our Heavenly Father. It is written, and it is final... whether one believes it or not.

We can live limited lives in unbelief and ignorance like those in the world.

We can also live heavenly lives empowered by the very Holy Spirit that gave birth to Jesus and anointed Him.

The knowledge of God's Word gives us understanding, and with godly understanding, we know what to do with every given situation that may come along.

Allow me to give you an example:

If a surgeon should cut himself by mistake, he may suffer a little bit of pain, but not fear.

Why?

Because he or she has learned just how the body works.

The surgeon understands what is happening and knows what to do about it.

Fear comes from not understanding a situation, and lack of understanding comes from a lack of knowledge.

Now, take a little child in the same situation.

Not knowing what is happening or what to do, he or she panics and blows everything out of proportion.

The child **suffers from not only pain, but also from fear.**

A lack of understanding in any troubled time gives room to fear.

Three months after I was healed 1n 1983, I was attacked with all of the symptoms of the migraine headaches that I was delivered from.

It really took me by surprise.

However, the word inside my heart checked and calmed me.

Consequently, I did not fear. (An unusual experience by the way...)

At that time I still had unused medicine in my home and I remember clearly being tempted to use it.

But I chose to resist the evil one, and the symptoms that racked my body with pain.

I had to resist for some hours, but when I decided that I would never take medicine again, I was instantly set free and healed.

A feeling of joy and ecstasy flooded throughout my entire being like a thousand diamonds being poured into it!

Yes, we do have emotions and feelings, and yes, we do have to deal with the evil things that take place in the earth on a daily basis.

But, we have the power from the throne room of God to defeat the same temptations as Jesus did.

Our bodies are on the earth and are exposed to the "world" (that is, the fallen realm of sinful man, the devil, and his demons).

But they are not subject to the world.

They are governed and empowered by our spirits and the Holy Spirit. We have become one in spirit with Christ.

The more you and I read the Word and get to know and understand God and His healing power, the less fear we have in tough situations.

Many beautiful Christians have died young. Others have suffered continual ill health.

Why?

Because of a lack of knowledge about God's Word concerning the soul.

The Bible describes us as being made up of three parts; **spirit, soul, and body.** (See 1 Thessalonians 5:23).

The spirit is that part of us that has come directly from God Himself. It is the part of us that is most like our Father, and it is where we commune with God.

The soul is the communication center between the spirit realm (heavenly places) and the natural; and/or the spirit and the body. The makeup of the soul is comprised of the mind, the will, and the emotions.

The body is simply the housing unit for the soul.

If the devil is able to paralyze the soul, he is then able to cut all power and communication between the spirit of man and his body.

Therefore, man becomes isolated from God's direct help.

Of course, God will try other ways to communicate with us like through a fellow believer, or our memory (if it is free to operate), or through reading the Bible.

(For further insight in this area, I encourage you to seek wise counsel from the elders of your church. It is a fascinating subject.)

We have learned to trust in physicians and medicines, especially during the last century.

The trust of our forefathers in God is now directed to the creation, that is, man instead of God the Creator.

Because of the fear of disease and pain, we rely on the physicians.

In turn, they have received much wealth and authority. To many, the physician has become their god.

However, the Word of God does not tell us to go to a physician or take medicine, but it does tell us to go to the elders if we are sick and they will anoint us with oil. It also says that the prayer of faith will heal us. (James 5:14-16)

A little dangerous?

Only if you have your faith in the medicine or physician.

The scriptures advise us to seek the counsel of the elders, who will help us and agree with us in prayer. The prayer and counsel restores the soul, and then the body of the believer receives the restoration power from the throne room of God.

If you should become ill, what should you do?
Look what the Bible says concerning sickness and healing.

Let's go to the book of James (Ch.5,vs. 14-16). *"Is any sick among you? Let him call for the elders of the church; and let them pray over him, anointing him with oil in the name of the Lord. And the prayer of faith shall save the sick., and the Lord shall raise him up; and if he have committed sins, they shall be forgiven him. Confess your faults one to another, and pray one for another, that ye may be healed."*

I enjoy counseling the sick because it is the ministry that God has given to me within the body of Christ.

Most people that come to me for prayer either believe that God heals, or that God cares for the sick and troubled.

Both of these statements are true, and the words, **"you were healed by the wounds of Jesus,"** are the truth.

False doctrines, or part truths, allowed in the mind because of the lack of knowledge can cause a believer to be full of fear and doubt.

In my ministry, I first deal with the fear and doubt by the Word of God, and then I lead the person through a prayer of reconciliation to God and His power. The result is that the person receives his or her healing and is freed from confusion.

Most of those who have been deeply wounded need a follow-up teaching on healing.

Therefore, I take them to scriptures in the Bible, **in order to ensure clear doctrine**, so that the illness or symptoms are not able to return.

Because of the fear of suffering, we find ourselves compelled to act.

Never act when compelled by fear.

For by doing this, we reverence the devil and his system.

All of our actions should be based on love, because God is love.

There is no more fear when we walk with God, for it is written that perfect love casts out fear.

Now, I would like you to ask yourself a question... What is my first reaction to my need?

Is it fear?

The answer should be, of course, the Word of God.

It is written that *God has not given us a spirit of fear, but of power, love, and a sound mind.* (2 Timothy 1:7)

Unfortunately, as I said earlier, many beautiful Christians have died before their time because of the counsel of men.

Without faith we cannot receive the promises.

Without faith we cannot be born again.

It is written, *"By grace through faith you are saved,"* and it is the same with healing. (Not to mention every other promise.)

Healing is a gift.

A gift given by grace.

But through faith you receive (or accept) this wonderful gift.

I know that you now have many questions, but please bear with me.

Please don't risk your life on vain philosophy, which may be no more than the mere counsel of men.

Ask God for understanding.

Next time you have an immediate need, pray and agree together on a scripture.

Ask God for wisdom and how to pray, and what to pray for.

Then act according to the Holy Spirit's leading and the Word of God.

Do not act in fear or doubt, for it is written that when you pray, **believe!**

When we choose to trust in God's Word, fear leaves us, and the voice of doubt is stopped.

The Word of God is the sword of the Holy Spirit (Ephesians 6:17).

So use the Word of God, which brings knowledge over fear.

Use it to stop the mouth of the devil and all his demons, and even the mouth of doubting men and all their vain philosophies.

"But let him ask in faith,

nothing wavering."

- James 1:6 -

Chapter Four

What is Faith?

"Now faith is the substance of things hoped for, the evidence of things not seen."

- Hebrews 11:1-

This quotation from the New Testament answers many questions concerning biblical faith.

Let us look at this scripture together. *"Faith is the substance* (something tangible) *of things hoped for, the evidence* (realization) *of things not seen* (by the natural eye)."

You and I have desires, and we hope (not wish) that some day our desires will materialize.

Without hope (or earnest expectation), we would give up.
The Bible tells us that hope is the anchor of our faith.

Faith gives substance to the desires that we hope for, and faith is the realization of our desires that cannot be seen by the natural eye.

The Gospel of Mark (ch.11 vs. 23) states that when we pray, we should believe (trust God) that we have received them (the things or desires), and we shall have them.

This scripture tells us how to *apply* our faith, or belief, whereas, the scripture in Hebrews (11:1) describes what faith is.

I can remember having a desire to be used by God as far back as my teenage years.

However, it wasn't until January 1988 that I started to prepare for the ministry. In other words, **my desires had no substance until then**.

Now, if I had never acted upon the Word of God, that is, the God-given visions and desires of my heart, I would have had nothing to show for it today.

Faith also gives substance to prayers that need immediate results.

Remember the scripture (Mark 11:23): *"When you pray, believe that you receive them and you shall have them."*

Notice that in this scripture, there is no time limit.

A good example is the prayer of salvation, or the prayer to be "born again."

How long does it take to be born again?

No time at all.

It's as quick as the revelation quickens the unbeliever and his or her response to trust God's word.

Well, it is the same for any other prayer of faith.

Both involve the simplicity of trusting God's Word in any area of life.

My wife Angelika and I, were once in a situation where we did not have enough gas to drive to church and back home again.

We also had an invitation to meet a museum owner that afternoon who lived some fifty miles out of our way.

(You can imagine how embarrassed we felt that morning.)

However, we chose to ask God about the situation, and the scripture about praying and believing came to mind.

I remember answering God with the question of what we should believe for, and was inspired with the idea of someone coming up to us and handing us one hundred German Marks, (about $60 USD at that time.)

Angelika and I decided to trust God for this provision and we drove to church.

Everyone who came up to us was a potential helper, because we believed what we had prayed.

In addition to our prayer, we agreed not to speak to anyone about our need, even if someone had brought up the subject.

After the morning's service ended, we found ourselves with no other choice but to head to our car.

Somewhat pensively, we headed to the parking lot which happened to be about a hundred yards down the road from the church.

The only thing left to do was to **encourage each other by God's Word and just keep on believing.**

What Is Faith?

I remember the weather being extremely cold, and we were dressed appropriately.

My wife was wearing her mink coat, and I was wearing a full-length suede coat.

In addition, we were driving a silver metallic colored Jaguar so we surely did not look like we were in need.

However, on our way to the car, we heard our names being called out.

As we turned, we were shocked to see a friend running up to us!

She stopped in front of us and, still panting for breath, asked us not to be offended with the question that she was about to ask.

We assured her that we wouldn't. So she blurted out, "Is everything okay?"

Keeping to our promise of not even suggesting that we were in need, we assured her that all was well.

Then she explained that God had told her to give us one hundred marks.

These words were certainly sweet to our souls!

We told her that she had definitely heard from God and after handing us the money, she went off skipping with delight because she had heard from God.

She was more excited than us!

The scripture, *"It is more blessed to give that to receive,"* (Acts 20:35) certainly came to mind and we praised Jesus for the miracle!

Why have I shared that precious moment with you?

Because we learned a very valuable lesson from it.

We saw first hand the power of the Word of God in action.

Our trust in God's Word brought us to prayer and not panic in a time of embarrassment and need.

Our faith, coupled with God's wisdom, brought results.

In other words, our **trust in God was the substance: our actions, the evidence.**

Together, they became the faith that we were going to receive what we had prayed for.

Though the needed 100 German Marks was not yet seen in the natural, our "faith eyes" directed by the scriptures, saw our Christian friend handing us the money.

Our prayers were given substance when we decided to act upon the word given by the Holy Spirit and directed by the Holy Spirit.

The faith we have been talking about is a God given gift to you and I.

It is a gift given so that we may learn to trust in God and His heavenly kingdom.

Most of us have been trusting in ourselves and the things of this world, but the Holy Spirit has come to teach us to trust and rely upon the supernatural power of God over the natural elements that we are used to.

As we learn to trust God, we will find ourselves falling in love with Him, for without trust we are unable to have a basis for love.

By the way, the word "trust" and the word "faith" are often interchangeable throughout the Bible.

How do we get faith?

The Bible tells us that **faith has been given to each one of us.** (Romans 12:3)

Also, it tells us that *faith comes by hearing and hearing by the Word of God.* (Rom. 10:17).

Note here that this scripture does not say that faith comes by hearing the Word of God.

No, hearing comes by the Word and faith comes by hearing.

Hearing what?

Hearing the voice of the Holy Spirit.

Finally, let us restate the scripture.

Faith comes by hearing the voice of the Holy Spirit, and hearing the Holy Spirit comes by (through) the Word of God.

This scripture definitely points to reading and knowing God's Word and the person of the Holy Spirit. And knowing the Holy Spirit is the most wonderful experience of all.

Chapter Five

The Holy Spirit

"And I will pray the Father, and He shall give you another Comforter, that He may abide with you forever; even the Spirit of truth..."

- John 14:16-17 -

The Holy Spirit is continually helping us as we walk according to the scriptures and according to His leading.

In fact, He will take the scriptures on healing and apply them to our body, mind, and emotions.

However, there is an enemy out there who loves to attack the souls of believers. That enemy is the devil and his cohorts.

Like a pack of wolves they come to rob, kill, and destroy knowing that if the believer can be cut off, the believer can become sick.

Consequently, if the believer does not seek help, they can lose their earthly body and their ministry will come to an end.

Fear not though, our Eternal Helper, the Holy Spirit has been given to us to remedy our helplessness!

He is a Spirit who gives us power, who gives us love, and who gives us a sound mind!

Lack of fellowship with the Holy Spirit can cause us to misunderstand the message that He gives us from the throne room of God.

We must learn to listen to the still small voice of the Holy Spirit.

Also, we must realize that **He is a person** and can be grieved if we do not know how to act in His presence.

Like it is in a marriage, we have to learn to keep an open relationship which can only be accomplished through practice and the passage of time.

We must also learn to spend time with the Holy Spirit knowing that any form of sin will grieve Him.

God forbid that we live in sin, for **we absolutely need the Holy Spirit's counsel and help to be victorious Christians.**

The Holy Spirit is also the one who reveals the healing of Jesus to us and applies it to our wounds. He is the power force that energizes our bodies.

Throughout the Bible, we see the Father, His Word (Jesus), and the Holy Spirit all working together as one.

The Father speaks the Word, which is Jesus, and the Holy Spirit is the creative force behind that which is spoken.

Jesus tells us in Acts, chapter one, verse eight, *"That when the Holy Spirit comes upon us, we would receive power."*

Romans 8:11 tells us that the Spirit of Him who raised Jesus from the dead **dwells in you**, and that He, the Holy Spirit, will also give life to your mortal bodies.

Therefore, I encourage you to acknowledge the Holy Spirit and His precious presence in your life.

In fact, you should do it this very moment.

Simply reverence the Lord and invite the Holy Spirit to reveal Jesus and His power of healing to you.

Finally, keep thanking your Heavenly Father as you await the presence of the Holy Spirit and His supernatural power to energize your body and mind.

Speaking of the manifestation of the Holy Spirit, one of the ways He reveals Himself to us is by experiencing an intense heat moving throughout the body.

At that moment, you may feel like going into unconsciousness, or you may break out in a sweat.

Do not fear, but receive His love and healing with thanksgiving.

He is the one who created us from the beginning of time.

(Thank you Jesus for bringing us back to the Father and His love.)

Now, we need to acknowledge His help.

Always remember that as we are the body, Jesus is the head, and that He is God.

Remember, that we were created in His image by Him and that He has no beginning nor end.

Of course, we have a beginning, for He made us.

God has given Himself to us in a special relationship, like marriage, but He is still the one and only God... Father, Son, and Holy Spirit.

My philosophy, before I made a decision to trust in Jesus as Lord and Savior, was to try my best not to sin but that it was impossible to avoid sinning on a regular basis.

I also thought that it was not so bad to do little sins, and if some big ones did occur, well... God would understand.

Unfortunately, that philosophy was taking me to the grave with a one-way ticket.

If it wasn't for a visitation from Jesus, and the inspiration of the Holy Spirit, I would have given up altogether.

You see, I had been brought up in a Christian home with the best schooling, and had no excuse for my newly developed unethical behaviors.

However, I knew deep down in my subconscious that I alone was to blame for my actions.

I desperately needed some answers and help before I went too far.

In the aforementioned visitation, Jesus appeared to me and said these words, "You can walk even as I walked."

With that statement, I knew that He was calling me to walk *with* Him and that it was possible to walk a path without sin.

I also knew that it could only be done through His power.

He Himself demonstrated this fact with His own life while on the earth.

The visitation itself reassured me that **He was alive and was willing to help me.**

You can imagine the precious hope that flooded my soul as the desire to follow Jesus was ignited.

I found out later that the power that worked through Jesus was the Holy Spirit and that we are not alone to work out our salvation, but the **Holy Spirit and the Word of God is with us and in us to defeat the power of sin** in every area of our lives.

Praise God! Praise Jesus!

Listen to Him for instructions.

We must learn to recognize the voice of the Holy Spirit to be able to walk by faith, knowing scripture is not just for knowledge's sake, but it is power and life to us who walk as sons and daughters of God.

As sons and daughters, we are called to live here on earth to glorify Jesus and with the direct power from God, we are invincible.

We must however, remain in open communication with the Father.

That is why Satan will try everything to cut off the line of communication.

One of the things that can cut the line of communication and grieve the Holy Spirit is the power of the tongue.

The book of James warns us of it.

Chapter three tells us that the tongue is a fire and a world of iniquity. It defiles the whole body and is full of deadly poison.

We are told that we bless God, and at the same time, we curse men that have been made in the likeness of God.

This is why we need Jesus and the power of the Holy Spirit.

Alone, we don't stand a chance.

I found out later that the power that worked through Jesus was the Holy Spirit and that we are not alone to work out our salvation, but the Holy Spirit and the Word of God is with us and in us to defeat the power of sin in every area of our lives.

Praise God! Praise Jesus!

As human beings, we find it easier to speak negatively about a difficult situation than to stand on the Word and speak positively.

We have to deal daily with our pride (what people think of us, or what they may say about us).

We all have a choice to speak as Jesus would, or to hold our peace.

In conclusion, remember that the Holy Spirit is a person, and He is with you forever.

Ever since I have invited Him into my daily walk, my life has been truly energized. My confidence and trust in God's Word has increased.

Being aware of the Holy Spirit's presence, (or acts), will help you and ultimately keep you in touch.

Chapter Six

Receive Your Healing Now!

"Behold, Now is the accepted time, behold, now is the day of salvation."

-2 Corinthians 6:2 -

God's Word says that we were healed by His stripes (the wound's on Jesus' body), and that He bore our pains (mental and physical), and took our sicknesses.

Do you believe in this?

Can you trust these words with your life?

We trust men with our lives and we trust ourselves, but will you trust God with your life?

It is the first step in the journey of healing.

Scriptures like 2 Chronicles 16:12 warn us to be alert to the counsel of God.

King Asa, one of the good kings of Judah, pleased God with many worthy acts until he chose the counsel of physicians over God's. It is written that King Asa died from the result of his choice.

The scriptures: *"By His stripes you were healed"* (1 Peter 2:24), and *"He took our pains and carried our sicknesses"* (Matthew 8:17) still remain powerful **for those who decide to trust in them with their whole heart, soul, mind, and strength.**

Jesus quoted the First Commandment to His followers, which reads... "to love God with all your heart, all your soul, all your mind, and all your strength." (Matthew 22:37.)

We can understand by this commandment that God does not accept partial belief and worship. He demands total commitment, and yet with great understanding God awaits our reaction to His gift of love.

That is the gift of His son Jesus Christ.

If we trust in the counsel of man, should we expect God to be pleased and help us anyway?
Let us please God with our faith and turn away from the ways of the world around us.

I'd like to give you an example of a struggle and eventual victory in this area.

It is the story of a certain lady in her thirties who underwent an operation to remove cancer from her ovaries. At the time she was not walking with God, and didn't know the healing scriptures of the Bible.

Her physician told her that the operation would remove all chances of having another child. However, in desperation she decided to go through with the operation.

Some years afterward, the lady noticed that the previous symptoms were returning and signs of the cancerous cells were becoming visible.

But that time, she trusted God for her healing because she had **learned the scriptural promises in the Bible.**

After prayer and the laying on of hands, she received her healing and the complications that she was having stopped.

I suggest that now is the time for you to read all of the scriptures that you can base your faith upon.

In fact, read them out loud and listen carefully to what you are reading.

Always use the Word of God in all prayers, **because it is the sword of the Holy Spirit.** (Ephesians 6:17).

Imagine yourself as a child of a King and the privilege you would have by being born into his family. As a newborn, you would not know your rights, but you would still have the inheritance.

As you grow into a child, you have to be tutored.

Well, right now, the Word of God is your inheritance, and the Holy Spirit is your tutor.

It is written, *"Ask and it will be given to you, seek and you shall find, knock and it will be opened unto you."*

Ask the Holy Spirit to reveal the answers to all of your questions.

Do not be angry or fear. John 14:26 says, *"But the Comforter (Helper), which is the Holy Ghost, whom the Father will send in my name, he shall teach you all things, and bring all things to your remembrance whatsoever I have said to you."* And, *"...when He, the Spirit of truth, is come, he will guide you into all truth..."* (John 16:13).

Remember, God has delivered you from the power of darkness, and translated you into the kingdom of his Son. (Colossians 1:13).

It is written in the book of Hebrews: ***"Ye are come unto mount Sion, and unto the city of the***

living God, the heavenly Jerusalem, *and to an innumerable company of angels, to the general assembly and church of the firstborn, which are written in Heaven,* ***and to God the judge of all,*** *and to the spirits of just men made perfect,* ***and to Jesus the mediator of the new covenant,*** *and to the blood of sprinkling, that speaketh better things than that of Abel."*

We don't have to leave this earth to be with God. We are already seated with Him at His right hand. Jesus sits there and **we are His body**.

We have been raised together and sit together with Christ in heavenly places (Ephesians 2:6), at the right hand of God the Father; far above all principality and powers and might and dominion, and every name that is named, not only in this age but in the age to come. (Eph. 1:20-21).

In heavenly places there is no pain and sorrow, no death and no evil.

All evil was cast out of the presence of God.

We, however, have come to that place.

By grace (not by the works of man, for grace is unmerited favor) **through faith.**

Here we come back to the word of faith again.

Remember what the Holy Bible says about faith?

I explained it earlier when I said that faith is "to trust in" or "rely upon."

Yours and my faith should be in the now. That is, in heavenly places where we rule and reign with Jesus.

I remember when I preached this message not long ago in a Methodist church. I told the congregation that the Holy Spirit would demonstrate, right before their eyes, that **we can receive our healing in the now; ...and then I added, "if we only believe."**

The first person that I was called to lay hands upon was a crippled lady of about sixty years of age. She hadn't walked for years.

After the prayer of faith, the lady stood up and started walking around the room!

I didn't even have to encourage her, for the power of the Holy Spirit regenerated her body right before our eyes.

You can only guess what happened to all the others that came for healing.

You must understand something, we are no longer subject to time, if we walk by faith.

By the faith that is according to God's Word, we are in the throne room of Heaven seated at the right hand of God in Christ Jesus.

In Heaven, the time is always NOW! Heaven is not subject to time as is the earth.

On earth, we are used to a time frame. Therefore, to the natural mind, everything must take time.

However, our measuring rod is God's Word, and not the norm of this world.

Allow me to illustrate.

A Japanese student whom I met during night classes at Bible college had wrecked her car.

She even suffered back injuries from the accident, and was fearing the worse case scenario because of a numbness that was within her right leg.

Her physician took X-rays, and could do little to relieve the constant pain.

The students and the teacher all prayed for the Japanese girl's healing.

However, I noticed that the prayers were not in the "now" and that she received little or no comfort.

My heart went out to her with the compassion of my Savior.

Upon leaving the classroom, I explained the position of my faith in God's Word and told her that **she could receive her healing right away.**

I could see that she was receiving my counsel so after the laying on of hands and the prayer of faith, she experienced an immediate surge of power going throughout her body.

Guess what?

The pain and weariness left her right there and then. Glory to God!!

Afterwards, her physician verified the healing with further X-rays.

Praise God for His healing for us is right now!!!

In the Old Testament, we hear the teachings about Daniel and how long it took for his prayers to be answered. That is a true story because it is God's Holy Word, but we now have the New Testament and are under **better promises and in a far better place.**

We are born of God.

The prophets of old were not born of the Holy Spirit, but were simply empowered by Him to fulfill God's will.

However, that same Spirit of God now dwells in us.

It was said by Jesus that John the Baptist was the greatest of all the prophets, and yet He also said the least in the kingdom of God is greater than John. (See Matthew 11:11).

He told His disciples to cast out demons, to lay hands upon the sick, and if they should drink any deadly thing it would not harm them.

Missionaries have had to rely upon these words daily,

It is important to remember that they are the same for us. Remember that **the devil is real**.

Therefore, it is necessary to address Satan and bind (stop) him in the name of Jesus. (Matthew 18:18).

According to John 10:10, he comes only to steal, kill, and destroy, but God is equally real and has all power to heal, rebuke, and recreate.

Ephesians 6:12 - 13 says, *"For we do not wrestle against flesh and blood, but against principalities, against powers, against spiritual hosts of wickedness in heavenly places. Therefore, take up the whole armor of God, that you may be able to withstand the evil day, and having done all, to stand."*

We are not to war against each other, but the fight is against the devil and his demons.

Anything that opposes the Bible is from the devil. What do we do with the devil?

"Resist him and he will flee from you." (James 4:7).

How do we resist the devil if we have already allowed sickness and fear to enter our bodies and minds?

Even without another believer nearby, you can receive your healing and freedom.

First, submit yourself to the Lord and ask Him to forgive you, then bind Satan under the scriptures. (Scriptures like Matthew 18:18.)

Just say, "In the name of Jesus Christ, I bind you Satan and the demon forces that are attacking me. **You have no legal power over me**."

Then, command fear and doubt to leave your mind and proclaim the scripture... "God has not given me a spirit of fear, but of power, love, and a sound mind." (2 Timothy 1:7).

Dwell on this scripture until you believe that you are free.

Now, bring the blood of Jesus before the Heavenly Father to **cancel all accusations** from the devil, for the blood paid for **all** of your sins.

This is serious, for **Satan is the accuser of the brethren and you must fight his spirits with the Word of God**.

The Word is the sword of the Holy Spirit.

The devil has been defeated and disarmed and made to be a public spectacle. (Colossians 2:15).

Remember what I said earlier, **you and I are sons and daughters of God here on earth for the purpose of ruling and reigning in the name of Jesus. Therefore, we are no longer subject to the kingdom of darkness**, but we are in the kingdom of Heaven and God.

The world of sin and death is the kingdom of darkness where we once lived under it's rules.

But the kingdom that we now live in, through Jesus Christ, is righteousness, peace, and joy in the Holy Spirit. (Romans 14:17).

We now live in Christ and no longer have to suffer the penalty of sin which is suffering and death.

When Jesus loosed a woman from a spirit of infirmity that had kept her bent over for eighteen years, she was immediately made well. (Luke 13:11).

Jesus declared, *"But if I cast out demons with the finger of God, than surely the Kingdom of God has come upon you."* (Luke 11:20).

Beware of any fear-motivated thoughts. This is another way that Satan's devils work. Do not dwell on them, but command them to go from you and to never return.

God has given us faith as a shield to ward off the devil's attacks. Use your faith, for faith quenches all the fiery darts of the wicked one. (Ephesians 6:14).

At this point, we should address the pain or sickness in the name of Jesus, naming the disorder, and telling it that you have chosen to rely on God's Word.

Do you still have pain or symptoms?

If so, there is something stopping your healing.

Remember, it is written that you were healed and God cannot lie, in fact, it is impossible for Him to lie.

Furthermore, command everything that is not of God to leave you now.

Do you know what time it is in Heaven?

It is NOW!!!

It is written that **now** is the acceptable time; behold **now** is the day of salvation.

You must command all pain to leave you and to not return.

You must be violent with demonic forces, until they learn who has the authority.

Jesus said to His disciples that all authority had been given to Him, and He gave it to us through the use of His name. (Matthew 28:18, Luke 10:19)

Let us read Mark 11:22-24. ***"Have faith in God. For assuredly I say to you, whoever says to this mountain, 'Be removed and be cast into the sea,' and does not doubt in his heart, but believes that those things he says will come to pass, he will have whatever he***

says. Therefore I say to you, whatever things you ask when you pray, believe that you receive them, and you will have them,"

Let's take this passage step by step:

"Have faith in God," means to trust in and act upon the Word of God.

The words, *"whoever says to this mountain, 'be removed and be cast into the sea,"* encourages us to speak to the sickness or symptom in the name of Jesus.

The words, *"and does not doubt in his heart but believes,"* tells us to stand in faith and not to doubt what is written in the Bible no matter what comes against our faith.

Remember, we are also told to bring every thought into captivity to the obedience of Christ. (2 Corinthians 10:5).

At a Full Gospel Business Men's meeting, a lady came to me for prayer.

She looked to be about eight months pregnant, so I asked her what I should pray for..., "perhaps for her baby?"

She told me that there was no baby, but rather that it was a very large tumor in her abdomen.

You can imagine how surprised I was, if not a little embarrassed.

However, instead of listening to the circumstances, I listened to the voice of the Holy Spirit who assured me that the healing of a headache was the same for Him as the healing of a tumor.

I laid my hands upon her, cursed the tumor, and set her free in the name of Jesus.

(Incidentally, I was reminded of how Jesus had cursed the fig tree and it withered.)

I will never forget this incident because the lady fell forward and not backwards. In fact, she fell on top of me like a ton of bricks, bringing both of us to the floor.

Again, a little embarrassing..., but wonderful because of the power of God.

Can I tell you that there are witnesses today who personally saw that lady walk away with a baggy dress dragging the floor?

She was instantly healed and delivered!

Praise the Lord.

To witness the miracles of God is an eye opener to the truth, and the truth is the good news of Jesus Christ.

Anyone who knows the scriptures well, knows that the devil and his demons were still active during the time of Jesus and the early church. Acts 10:38 reads... *"How God anointed Jesus of Nazareth with the Holy Spirit and with power, who went about doing good and healing all who were oppressed by the devil."*

This points out that sickness was a result of demonic oppression.

Many other scriptures portray demonic activity in the early church.

Paul suffered from a *"messenger from Satan,"* and he called it, *"a thorn in the flesh."* (2 Corinthians 12:7).

We are still in the Day of Salvation, and Satan and his devils are still free to roam the earth.

Just a side note: We must not forget to command all demons to the Abyss (the bottomless pit.)

We have angels to minister to us for everything (Hebrews 1:14.) They will come to our rescue whenever they hear the Word of God on our behalf.

In conclusion, here is my prescription:

Bind all doubts and fears in the name of Jesus and cast them to the Abyss where God sent the rebellious angels before the flood.

After the prayer of faith, if symptoms still persist, you must speak to the sickness or symptom and command it to leave you and be cast into the Abyss as well.

Keep your confession of being healed.

According to your faith, be healed and get going for God.

And finally, to seal the deal, do something that demonstrates your faith and follow that up with a testimony of God's miracle working power.

"Wherefore seeing we also

are compassed about

with so great a cloud of witnesses,

let us lay aside every weight,

and the sin

which doth so easily beset us,

and let us run with patience

the race that is set before us..."

- Hebrews 12:1 -

Chapter Seven

Avoiding Hindrances

*"Christ hath redeemed us from the curse of the
law, being made a curse for us... "*

- Galatians 3:13 -

A negative confession will keep you from receiving
your inheritance, which includes good health and
divine healing.

Not long ago I discovered a wonderfully simple
statement in the book of Isaiah.

It says that the inhabitant (of Mount Zion) will not
say, "I am sick." (Isaiah 33:24).

Remember, you and I as believers have entered
Mount Zion, **the city of the living God**, the
heavenly Jerusalem. (Heb. 12:22).

We are chosen to speak the words of our God,
nothing more and nothing less. Proclaiming our
salvation and healing is a statement of faith.

We are called not to be ashamed of the gospel of Christ, but to be bold before unbelievers.

By doing this, we put to shame the counsel of the ungodly, and **proclaim Jesus as Lord.**

There is a transformation and cleansing of our consciences when we are born of God through faith in the Word.

As sons and daughters of God, we want to be like our heavenly Father and like Jesus, our wonderful mediator and elder brother.

We may still sin, but we no longer enjoy evil things.

We gain a renewed conscience.

If you should sin, **it is written that the blood of Jesus cleanses you from all sin.** (1 John 1:7).

Did you know that God decided to reveal sin for what it really was?

Therefore, through Moses He gave the law.

Most of us have learned the Ten Commandments, but there was much more than just the Ten Commandments. In fact, **six hundred and thirteen laws came into effect to judge and reveal sin.**

If one studies these laws you will notice how God hates sin, and how sin and sickness are dealt with.

Obedience to the law of Moses brought blessings, but on the other hand, disobedience brought curses.

Among these curses were plagues, sickness, and pain. (Deuteronomy 28:15-68)

Original sin separated Adam and Eve from the protection of the Garden of Eden and the land became cursed. Consequently, pain was promised to Mankind. (Genesis 3:16-24).

In the New Testament, we find that **unbelief is counted as sin**.

"What is not faith is sin..." (Romans 14:23).

Evil fruits separate us from fellowship with God because those fruits amount to sin that has to be dealt with.

That's why Jesus died.

He died on the cross to restore our fellowship with God which was broken in the Garden of Eden.

Through Him, we are no longer under the curse of death, nor affected by the curse that harmed earth. Jesus became a curse that we could be loosed from the curses of the Law of Moses. (Genesis 3:13). And the blood of Jesus cleanses us from all sin, even if we should fall into unbelief.

Jesus dealt with sin so that we could be free from it's effects; i.e. sickness, poverty, fear, weakness, etc...

Sin is obviously a hindrance to our healing.

It is written that *if we confess our sins, He is faithful and just to forgive us our sins and to cleanse us from all unrighteousness.* (1 John 1:9).

If you really believe in the Word of God, you will change your life accordingly.

Of course, you need the power of the Holy Spirit to help you, which is one of the reasons why we have Him here with us on the earth.

Turn away from the things that do not line up with the Bible, and trust God for supernatural help. He, *"is a very present help in time of need."* (Psalm 46:1).

I now know that even a sarcastic remark can be used as an **open door** for pain and injury to enter.

For instance, I experienced a bad burn to my hand while I was ironing one day.

I had been arguing with my wife and judging her, when the iron fell off of the ironing board.

I caught it in midair... but I caught it by the hot metal part.

For some reason, I did not drop the iron right away, but carried it back to the ironing board while it seared into my skin. Maybe I was in shock, or maybe I was just still angry. Either way, my hand hurt terribly from deep burns.

(Thank God that the first words that came out of my mouth were, "Jesus, Jesus, Jesus," rather than...

Well, thank God for Jesus.)

While I called on His name, I heard a reply which challenged me. The words, "ask your wife for forgiveness," rang out in my conscience.

Obediently, I called out to my wife who was in the adjacent room. I asked her to please forgive me of my remarks.

She did, and went right on with what she was doing, not even being aware of my severe trial.

Then that inner voice told me to thank Him for my healing, and to carry on with what I was doing before the incident.

My hand was still burning, but the fear was gone.

With difficulty, I managed to dress and go out to the movie my wife and I had planned to attend.

On the way out of our house, Angelika noticed the burn but I told her that it was okay in Jesus' name. By that time she was used to my "funny" walk of faith and was amused.

I completely forgot about my burn on the way to the tram because the pain had left. I didn't even remember that I had burned myself until after the movie, but by then there were no visible signs of being burned at all!

Praise God.

Please hear what the Holy Spirit says to you through the description of this "happening" in my life. You too can have your healing right now, just as I received mine.

Notice that I listened to the Holy Spirit and acted quickly in obedience.

If I hadn't, the whole situation would have turned out to be very painful, and I wouldn't have learned this important lesson.

Similar injuries have occurred since, but each time I acted in faith, I received immediate relief and healing.

Remember not to judge others, especially a brother. When you judge, the Word tells us that we will be judged accordingly.

Forgive everyone.

If you find it difficult, then ask the Holy Spirit for He is here on the earth to help you.

Jesus forgave you while He hung on the cross in agony.

You must forgive to be forgiven.

The Bible tells us that unforgiveness breaks communication with our Heavenly Father. Unforgiveness can turn into bitterness and even hatred.

Jesus warned us, telling us that if we should hate our fellow man, it is as bad as to murder him.

The words, *"The road is narrow and the way is straight,"* come to mind as I write this warning.

We must be very careful with our thoughts. Meditating on the Word of God daily will keep us free.

We are still saved if we should sin, but we must confess our sins and ask the Holy Spirit to help us walk the walk of faith.

Faith has to be active because sin and the devil can cause us to fall into sickness or injury.

However, if we believe on Jesus, we have a Savior who is as close as the word of faith coming from our mouths. (Romans 10:8).

Arise my brother and sister. Arise and take your place beside the Father in Jesus' name.

Be bold and kick the devil out of your life with the name of Jesus and the Word of God.

Be violent with the evil one and his cohorts if they should try to stay.

Do not reason with anything that is contrary to the Word of God.

Do not look to the left, nor to the right, but to Jesus alone, *"the author and finisher of our faith."* (Hebrews 12:2). This is the Word of God.

Do not even look around you and judge God's Word with the circumstances of life, but rather judge the circumstances with the scriptures.

Even great men have faults, **but God cannot lie
or be tempted. It is that God who is your
Heavenly Father.**

He alone understands you and cares for you.

Trust in His Word.

Once we hear His voice, we know exactly what to do
in every given situation.

Those who walk in the spirit are sons of God.

We are called to die to ourselves and live in Christ,
which, by the way, is a daily commitment.

In other words, we go from glory to glory. That is,
less and less of ourselves, and more and more of
Jesus.

Now, command your body to line up with the Word
of God and function normally, naming whatever
part of your body that is affected, and test for pain.

If the pain is still there, even just a little, rebuke
again and cast it out in the name of Jesus.

Finally, ask the Holy Spirit to guide you in a prayer
of confession before the Father in Heaven. The
Holy Spirit will help you to repent, (turn away)
from the things that grieve Him and hinder your
recovery.

Remember, the blood of Jesus cleanses you continually from all sin for **He did not come to condemn, but to save. To save and to love you!!**

<u>*Chapter Eight*</u>

Thanking God and Rejoicing

"Enter into His gates with thanksgiving, And His courts with praise."

- Psalm 100:4 -

Thank God for your freedom, the work of the cross, and the resurrection of Christ.

Allow the Holy Spirit to help you seek His guidance.

Now thank God for the healing, your healing, that Jesus paid for when He went to the cross.

In fact, ask the Holy Spirit to reveal your healing to you right here and now.

Remember to keep thanking God for Jesus, who healed you by His wounds.

From now on, remember to **thank God daily** for your healing and good health.

I believe that you have heard the voice of the Holy Spirit throughout this book.

The Word of God is now powerful within you and your spirit is excited.

I believe with all of my heart that you are already feeling better.

It is written that *you shall know the truth and the truth shall make you free.* (John 8:32).

I know that you are experiencing the anointing of God as you read these words.

Praise your Heavenly Father for sending Jesus.

Let's read together from the book of Hebrews, starting at chapter 4:1 to cap all that I have had to say: *"Let us therefore fear, lest, a promise being left us of entering into His rest, any of you should seem to come short of it. For unto us was the gospel preached, as well as unto them: but the word preached did not profit them, not being mixed with faith in them that heard it. For we which have believed do enter into rest, as he said, As I have sworn in my wrath, if they shall enter into my rest: although the works were finished from the foundation of the world."*

Now is the acceptable time for your healing.

Not in five minutes, not in two, but "**now**" be healed.

Praise the Lord forever.

Jesus loves you.

My wife and I have not lived a painless life, but when we have allowed the enemy to afflict us, we have taken action according to the Word and cast Satan and his cohorts out. And every time, the healing of Jesus floods our bodies and minds, and we receive immediate comfort and strength.

So can you!

"If we confess our sins,

he is faithful and just

to forgive us our sins,

and to cleanse us

from all unrighteousness."

- 1 John 1:9 -

Chapter Nine

Recipes for Healing

"The Spirit of the Lord is upon Me, because He has anointed me to preach the gospel to the poor. He has sent me to heal the brokenhearted. To preach deliverance to the captives and recovery of sight to the blind, to set at liberty those who are oppressed. To preach the acceptable year of the Lord

- Luke 4:18-19 -

Do you really believe that Jesus the Christ has healed you?

If so, then go forth healed in faith and do what he says. If not, ask yourself why.

Then ask the Holy Spirit to reveal to you what the hold up is and what you should do about it...

Then do it!

Your remembrance of the testimonies of others and your own experience of how God worked in, through, and for you (and for those around you);

as well as His promises to you, will help to strengthen your faith.

Get others, the elders of your church, fellow believers, family, and friends to pray and help you to stand in faith against the evil one by doing that which you know is right.

Recognize, confront, and dispel your fears **with faith in the scriptures** followed by the appropriate actions and lifestyle.

One way to put all of this into practice is to do the following:

• **Confess your sins and receive the forgiveness and cleansing by the blood of Jesus.**

• **Receive the Bible as the only way to divine healing.**

• **Write down what you fear most and what the physician has to say about your condition.**

• **Write down the scriptures that promise healing and peace of mind.**

• **Choose which one you are going to trust... God's counsel or the counsel of man.**

• **Read all the scriptures that you can base your faith upon, out loud and listen carefully to them.**

• **Remind your Heavenly Father and yourself of His promises.**

• **Address Satan and bind him in the name of Jesus. (See Matthew 18:18).**

• **Bring the blood of Jesus before the Heavenly Father to cancel all accusations from the devil.**

• **Address the pain or sickness in the name of Jesus, naming the disease and telling it that the devil is powerless to help.**

• **Command everything that is not of God to leave you immediately. (Which includes all symptoms, diseases, demon forces, etc.)**

• **Finally, fellowship with the Holy Spirit, acknowledge His help, and listen to Him for instructions.**

After time, these should become second nature to you and you will begin to see the impossible become possible.

Let's look at them one last time...

• **Arise and put your faith into action.**

• **Do what the Holy Spirit tells you to do.**

• **Command your body to function normally.**

• **Take captive all imaginations under the Word of God.**

• **Thank God for your healing.**

• **Rejoice and tell others what God has done for you.**

- It's just that simple!

Prayer for Healing

"But He was wounded for our transgressions, He was bruised for our iniquities; The chastisement for our peace was upon Him, And by His stripes we are healed."

- Isaiah 53:5 -

What can I do now? The following is a prayer that can help you:

"Heavenly Father, in the name of Jesus I come before you.

Thank you for Jesus and all that He did for me. Thank you for cleansing me with His blood and buying me back from the devil.

Father, I bring to remembrance your Word. It is written that by the stripes of Jesus we were healed and that Jesus bore our pain and sicknesses.

Father, I chose to forgive everyone who has hurt me and disappointed me, and I loose them from my judgment.

Father, I choose to trust your Word above all other counsel.

Thank you for revealing the healing of Jesus to me and applying it to my body and mind.

I believe that now is the acceptable time for my healing.

Holy Spirit, please come along side me now and apply your healing by the stripes of Jesus to my body and mind.

Fill me with your power, now, in Jesus' name...

Satan, in the name of Jesus, I bind you now over my life! I break your power by the blood of Jesus. I command all symptoms to leave me know

Body and mind, I command you to be healed and line up pain free.

I am healed! I am delivered! I am cleansed by the blood of Jesus! Amen."

Also, the prayer of agreement has a special effect. We are exhorted to pray with our elders in the time of sickness. (James 5:14).

Scriptures of Life & Healing

"My people are destroyed for lack of knowledge..."

- Hosea 4:6 -

I would like to encourage you to speak out, confess, and memorize these and any other scriptures that promise healing and peace of mind. These are quoted from the King James version of the Bible.

"Who his own self bare our sins in his own body on the tree, that we, being dead to sins, might live unto righteousness, by whose stripes you were healed." (1 Peter 2:24).

"Himself took our infirmities and bare our sicknesses." (Matthew 8:17).

"Behold, now is the accepted time; behold, now is the day of salvation." (2 Corinthians 6:2).

"Who hath delivered us from the power of darkness, and hath translated us into the kingdom of his dear son." (Colossians 1:13)

"And having spoiled principalities and powers, he made a shew of them openly, triumphing over them in it." (Colossians 2:15).

"Even when we were dead in sins, hath quickened us together with Christ... And hath raised us up together, and made us sit together in the heavenly places in Christ Jesus." (Ephesians 2:56).

"Far above all principality, and power, and might and dominion, and every name that is named, not only in this world but also in that which is to come." (Ephesians 1:21).

"For God hath not given us the spirit of fear; but of power, and of love, and of a sound mind." (2 Timothy 1:7).

"There is no fear in love; but perfect love casteth out fear, because fear hath torment..." (1 John 4:18).

"Submit yourselves therefore to God. Resist the devil and he will flee from you." (James 4:7).

"Confess your faults one to another, and pray for one another, that ye may be healed." James 5:16).

"For the word of God is quick and powerful, and sharper than any two edged sword, piercing even to the dividing asunder of soul and spirit, and of joints and marrow, and is a discerner of the thoughts and intents of the heart." (Hebrews 4:12).

"... And the sword of the Spirit, which is the word of God." (Ephesians 6:17).

"For we wrestle not against flesh and blood, but against principalities, against powers, against the rulers of the darkness of this world, against spiritual wickedness in high places."
(Ephesians 6:12).

"For ye are all the children of God through faith in Christ Jesus." (Galatians 3:26).

"For the weapons of our warfare are not carnal, but mighty through God, to the pulling down of strongholds." (2 Corinthians 10:4).

"For the kingdom of God is not in word, but in power." (1 Corinthians 4:20).

"Unto him who loved is and washed us from our sins in his own blood, and hath made us kings and priests unto God and his Father..."
(Revelation 1:5-6).

"By ye shall receive power, after that the Holy Spirit has come upon you; and you shall be witnesses unto me...." (Acts 1:8).

"Go ye, therefore, and preach the gospel..."
(Mark 16:15).

"And these signs shall follow them that believe. in my name they will cast out devils; they shall speak with new tongues; they shall take up serpents; and if they drink any deadly thing, it shall not hurt

them; they shall lay hands on the sick and they will recover." (Mark 16:17).

"Now, faith is the substance of things hoped for, the evidence of things not seen." (Hebrews 1:1).

"... faith cometh by hearing, and hearing by the word of God." (Romans 10:17).

"But without faith it is impossible to please him (God)." (Hebrews 11:6).

"For we walk by faith, not by sight." (2 Corinthians 5:7).

"But let him ask in faith, nothing wavering." (James 1:6).

"But be ye doers of the word, and not hearers only, deceiving your own selves." (James 1:22).

"Even so faith, if it hath not works, is dead, being alone." (James 2:17).

"Seest thou how faith wrought with his works, and by works was faith made perfect?" (James 2:22).

"For unto us was the gospel preached, as well as unto them; but the word preached did not profit them, not being mixed with faith in them that heard it." (Hebrews 4:2).

"For whatsoever is not of faith is sin."
(Romans 14:23).

"Behold, now is the accepted time; behold, now is the day of salvation." (2 Corinthians 6:2).

"But exhort one another daily while it is called 'Today..." (Hebrews 3:13).

"For he that has entered his rest, he also hath ceased from his works, as God did from his."
(Hebrews 4:10).

"But if the spirit of him who raised up Jesus from the dead dwell in you, he that raised up Christ from the dead shall also quicken your mortal bodies by his Spirit that dwelleth in you."
(Romans 8:11).

"I shall not die, but live and declare the works of the Lord." (Psalms 118:17)

"I say to you,

Arise,

take up your bed and walk..."

\- Luke 5:24 -

<u>Special Bonuses For You:</u>

Visit <u>YouWereHealed.com</u> and sign in to read more from Eric Holzapfel and readers like you.

More teaching!
More testimonies!
More miracles!
More opportunities to see God at work today!

Share your testimony. Make new friends.

Get prayer for your specific situation and concerns.

Get extra copies of this book to distribute to those who really need it.

Interact with Eric in our online community.

Book Eric for speaking gigs.

Trade with others in our private marketplace.

And much, much more!

Join today for FREE!

<u>https://YouWereHealed.com</u>